C000186387

The Doctc

Venous L__g

Prevention & Treatment
By Kenneth Wright in consultation with
Alan Neil, Liza Ovington PhD and Dr.Louis Grondin.

Some content adapted, with thanks from the following organizations: CAWC (Canadian Association of Wound Care), WOCN (Wound Ostomy Continence Nurses) Association, the NPUAP (National Pressure Ulcer Advisory Panel)

A special thanks to the Physicians Association for Patient Education (PAPE) and the North American wound care nurses who provided direction and editing for this book

ISBN 978-1-896616-13-1
© 2015 Mediscript Communications Inc.

The publisher, Mediscript Communications Inc., acknowledges the financial support of the Government of Canada through the Book Publishing Industry Development Program (BPIDP) for our publishing activities.

Contact information:
mediscript30@yahoo.ca,
Tel: 800 773 5088
Fax: 800 639 3186 International
Tel: North America (519) 341 0211

Printed in Canada

Book and Front Cover design by:
Brian Adamson, www.AdamsonGraphics.net

IMPORTANT MESSAGE FROM THE PUBLISHER

This book provides sound, well accepted information to help the healing process and actually to prevent venous leg ulcers.

The treatments and specific prevention products and suggestions are broad in nature and are dependent upon the patient's health status. Only the physician or other health care professionals can accurately diagnose and assess the patient's condition.

Therefore, we emphasize that the information contained within this book is not a substitute for the patient's physician or other health care professional's advice and treatment. This book provides "generic" information on the overall principles of the treatment and prevention of venous leg ulcers.

A wide range of products are available, such as dressings, compression bandaging, compression stockings and skin care products as well as surgical procedures that can help patients. It is important to understand that your physician and other health care professionals are the only people who can make the right choices for the patient.

With this in mind, the publishers and authors disclaim any responsibility for any adverse effects resulting directly or indirectly from independently taking actions from the content of this book from the written information, from any undetected errors or from the reader's misunderstanding.

Ordering this book:
Retail Price: $5.95 - Discounts available for volume purchases.
Tel: 800 773 5088
Fax: 800 639 3186
Email: mediscript30@yahoo.ca
For other titles go to:
www.mediscript.net

YOUR DIRECTORY
Fill in these for easy reference

Family Physician's name:_____

Tel:_____ Emergency Tel: _____

Address _____

Wound Care Nurse's name: _____

Email _____ Tel:_____

Location _____

Physician Specialist:

Name _____ Type _____ Tel:_____

Name _____ Type _____ Tel:_____

Name _____ Type _____ Tel:_____

Pharmacy / Home care store: _____

Address _____

Tel:_____ email: _____

Compression stocking fitter's name:

_____

Emergency Contact information
(Hospitals / neighbors / cell phones)

Name _____ Tel:_____

Name _____ Tel:_____

Name _____ Tel:_____

Useful websites:

_____

_____

CONTENTS

Dear Reader,

Congratulations! You've just taken the first step in the journey to health and recovery from illness by acknowledging the importance of preventive measures on your part.

The single most important medication we as physicians can prescribe to our patients is an understanding of venous and circulatory disorders. Patients who understand their condition and the extent of its severity are best fitted to deal with any complications, setbacks and obstacles throughout the course of their lives. Knowledge, in this case, is truly power.

We are able to envision circulatory disease at a cellular and molecular level. We feel we are in the middle of the battleground and are finally able to take a hands-on approach, both in the management of illness and the prevention of cellular and organ dysfunction.

When it comes to venous disease, the single most effective intervention is regular daily exercise. When a venous patient decides not to exercise, he actually signs a contract with future complications of the disease, depending on his genetic background, obesity and basic state of health.

Daily exercise at any age regardless of the underlying complications will always help to kick-start the healing process.

This booklet provides an overview of the cause of venous ulcers, the treatments available for the condition and suggested key preventative measures such as the long-term use of compression stockings and lifestyle issues such as stopping smoking and good nutrition.

It is with great enthusiasm that I introduce this book on venous ulcerations.

Louis Grondin, M.D.
Medical Director
Cosmetic Laser and Vein Centre
Past President of the Society of Phlebology

INTRODUCTION

This is a self help booklet that can not only help you heal a leg ulcer faster but can provide you with tips in actually preventing a leg ulcer from developing. We like to think of this book as a "Reader's Digest" style of information, providing comprehensive, essential information in an easy to understand manner

A leg ulcer is a serious skin problem described best as an open wound which can even affect the soft tissues below the skin. Leg ulcers are responsible for a lot of discomfort, pain, emotional upset, absence from work and social disability. In other words venous leg ulcers can significantly impair the quality of life of those who suffer from them.

Leg ulcers are often looked upon as a chronic condition in which complete healing is difficult to attain and this should be a major motivator to prevent venous leg ulcers from occurring.

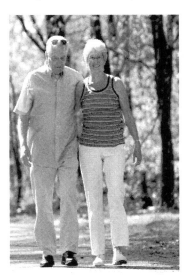

One statistic depicts half of the venous leg ulcer patients had a leg ulcer history spanning five to ten years, a third exceeding ten years. This shows venous leg ulcers to be a chronic and recurring problem

However new treatments, emotional support for patients, and patients learning to take on more responsibility in managing the condition are helping to turn things around.

There are three medically defined leg ulcers - arterial,

6

diabetic foot and venous. There are also skin ulcers with similar characteristics that can appear on other parts of the body which are called pressure ulcers or also known as bedsores or decubitus ulcers.

This book is only about the venous leg ulcer. "Venous" means associated with veins; "leg" is of course the location; ulcer is a medical term for a skin breakdown - essentially an open wound.

It is estimated that about 70%- 90% of all leg ulcers are caused by venous problems, consequently venous leg ulcers are the most common of all the leg ulcers. Studies have estimated that venous ulcers can occur in 1-2% of the population—it is estimated that there are well over half a million venous leg ulcer sufferers at any one time in North America.

Who should read this book:

The Patient: Venous leg ulcers are a "quality of life" issue. "Getting about", comfort, pain relief, embarrassment and other problems are all addressed in these pages. Carefully absorbing this information can help you get more involved in the treatment and self help prevention aspects.

The Caregiver: Helping a patient or family member with a leg ulcer or who is at risk of developing one can be so much easier if there is complete understanding. This booklet can be useful to refer to in tackling the problems.

The Health Care Worker: Venous leg ulcers can be demanding for you and the problems are sometimes compounded by poor patient cooperation and lengthy healing times. However this booklet can reinforce the medical team's advice and treatment measures and can eliminate problems of patients and caregivers forgetting important points. Health care workers or paraprofessionals have differing job titles according to the area or type of work performed. Such work titles include, personal support workers, home care aides, nurses aides, nursing assistants, personal care attendants, unlicensed assistive personnel, community health workers.

You may have been given this book from a health care professional such as a physician, nurse, educator, pharmacist or any other professional in order to empower you to have the extra confidence to work effectively in ensuring preventative and treatment actions are maintained.

Health Care Professionals: Counseling patients and caregivers take time and understandably, information is often forgotten or sometimes misunderstood. Consequently this book can be an invaluable educational aid for the professional in getting over and reinforcing the key health education messages.

An important point to emphasize to all readers is the appreciation that a patient should be managed holistically in that the whole patient should be treated as well as heal the ulcer and prevent recurrence. This means recognizing the patient's pain and suffering as well as providing the best possible wound care. It is not a stretch of reasoning to suppose that the healing rates of venous ulcers may improve if the energy now used by patients to cope with pain and suffering were used instead to heal their wounds.

The patient should try to be assertive and certainly not accept that pain and discomfort is the norm for a venous ulcer.

Caregivers and health workers should perhaps be more interventionist and become perhaps more skilled in asking the right questions to find out the extent of these emotional and comfort issues. There is always a danger in the medical profession to focus and analyze on the body (in this case the venous ulcer) and possibly trivializing the mind or the "feeling" experiences of the patient.

For whatever category of reader, this book is laid out so that you can reference a particular topic from the table of contents and obviously you can refer to that topic as stand - alone information that may satisfy your immediate information needs.

We have listed a number of websites for all levels of readers at the back of the book.

Finally, team effort between the medical profession, caregivers, health care workers and patient is the key to success. A patient should become actively involved in the management of the leg ulcer. The old adage "knowledge is power" is so appropriate when it comes to coping with a venous ulcer. Once you understand why a venous ulcer develops, and are aware of the warning signs as well as the rationale for the treatment process, you are more likely to become a true partner in the medical team effort.

KEY POINTS

- Venous Leg Ulcers are the most common form of leg ulcer by far.

- Venous ulcers can significantly affect quality of life.

- Venous ulcers can be chronic and recurring.

- Implementing prevention tips and adhering to treatment is vital.

WHAT ARE LEG ULCERS

We mentioned earlier that a venous leg ulcer is a skin problem usually characterized by an open wound. There are other conditions with a similar description which are not venous leg ulcers. So in case your physician mentions these other conditions let's take away any misunderstanding or ambiguity caused by the different terms:

Arterial leg ulcer: Caused by breakdown and disease of the arteries, the blood vessels carrying oxygenated blood to the leg and foot. This type occurs infrequently and the chances of healing this type of leg ulcer are very poor.

Diabetic foot ulcer: Due to both circulatory and nerve ending problems caused by the disease diabetes. These problems collectively create damaged skin and subsequent ulcers first by causing a loss of sensation within the foot whereby the patient does not feel pain. Subsequent damage to the skin can happen (an unnoticed tight shoe, an object lodged in the shoe, etc.). Then the impaired circulation of blood to the foot slows down the healing process and the ulcer can get worse.

Good foot care, diabetes management and careful treatment can improve this problem.

Pressure ulcers: There is a very common form of skin ulcer. These can be all over the body not just the leg. They are caused by sustained pressure on the skin cutting off the blood flow and causing the skin to break down and die. This happens mostly with people who are limited in how much they can move: bedridden patients, post surgical patients, paralyzed patients, etc. Other terms used for pressure ulcers are bedsores, decubitus ulcers, and pressure sores.

10

This book is about **venous leg ulcers** which occur just above the ankle, on the inside surface of the leg. Unlike arterial and diabetic leg ulcers where blood flow into the damaged area is impaired, the venous leg ulcer results from difficulties in the blood flow out of the affected area.

Here's a quick reference distinction between the three types of leg ulcers:

	Venous	Arterial	Diabetic
Location	Inside surface of leg Above the ankle	Top of foot or toes Above or below ankle	Toes Weight bearing surfaces Areas of friction
Shape	Irregular shape Shallow wound	Punched out appearance Deep "cliff" edge	Punched out Cliff edge/callous
Ulcer Surface Colour	Red / yellow drainage	Usually black Dry	Often or usually black Dry
Ulcer Size	Medium to large	Small	Small / very small
Edema / Swelling	Generalized lower leg	Localized around ulcer only (inflamation)	Absent
Leg / Foot Pulses	Normal	Reduced or absent	Present
Pain	Often present Worse with leg down Relieved with leg up	Often present Worse with leg up Relieved with leg down Night Pain	Often absent
Skin Staining	Usually	Rarely	Rarely
Ulcer Drainig Fluid	Yes	Rarely	Rarely
ABPI*	0.8 or above	Below 0.8	Unreliable

*ABPI is Ankle Brachial Pressure Index

CAUSES OF VENOUS LEG ULCERS

The underlying disease that can cause a venous leg ulcer is broadly labeled as "venous disease". "Venous" as we said earlier, relates to veins.

Understanding how this venous disease occurs will help you appreciate some of the treatment options described later in the book (notably compression bandages).

The following pie chart demonstrates the proportional incidence of venous diseases: as you can see by far the biggest health issue are varicose veins. Now, only a tiny percentage of varicose vein sufferers will develop leg ulcers but it's important to appreciate that varicose veins can be the first step in developing a venous leg ulcer. Sometimes the only problem for the patient with varicose veins is their unsightliness along with some aches and pains in the leg when that is the case, very little treatment, if any, is required.

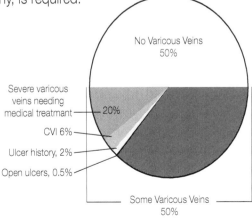

No Varicous Veins 50%

Severe varicous veins needing medical treatmant — 20%

CVI 6%

Ulcer history, 2%

Open ulcers, 0.5%

Some Varicous Veins 50%

The next serious step is the development of CVI (Chronic Venous Insufficiency) and this venous disease can be the stepping stone to a venous leg ulcer.

Looking at the big picture in North America more than 500,000 people are undergoing treatment right now. In fact 1-2% of the population has the underlying venous problem that can lead to a venous leg ulcer. And unfortunately, approximately two-thirds of those who have experienced one venous leg ulcer will eventually go on to develop at least one more.

An understanding of what causes venous leg ulcers can be a real help in preventing them or in helping them to heal. The ulcer is a symptom or a sign that not enough oxygen or nutrients are reaching the damaged skin area. To understand this you have to appreciate the basics of how blood flows throughout your body.

Your blood flow system

The flow of blood throughout your body is carried out by two types of blood vessels: arteries and veins.

Arteries carry blood rich in oxygen from the heart to all parts of the body. (Your body needs this oxygen for energy.) These arteries have thick muscular walls and can squeeze the blood onwards through their own contractions.

Veins, on the other hand, are thin walled and do not have muscles to pump the blood onwards. Their function is to return blood, which has given up its oxygen to the tissues, back to the heart.

The lack of muscles within the walls of the veins and the problems of pumping upwards (against gravity) make it quite a challenge for the veins to get the de-oxygenated blood back to the heart.

Unfortunately, the force generated by the heart cannot, unassisted, overcome the forces of gravity and drive the blood from the toes back to the brain.

Another mechanism is involved in which the calf muscles of the legs, when they contract, squeeze the deep veins and propel blood upwards. Downward flow of the blood is prevented by the presence of valves found at regular intervals in the deep veins. These valves divide the veins into sections, each valve forming a "floor" to support the blood above it.

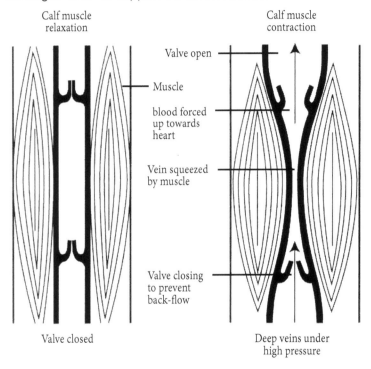

Calf muscle relaxation

Calf muscle contraction

Valve open

Muscle

blood forced up towards heart

Vein squeezed by muscle

Valve closing to prevent back-flow

Valve closed

Deep veins under high pressure

At the end of each heartbeat the valves in the veins close to stop the blood flowing backwards.

These veins are connected to one another by perforating veins which carry blood from the superficial vein to the deep veins. When the perforating vein meets the deep vein reverse flow is prevented by a one way valve.

Should these perforating vein valves fail, blood from t
vein system is forced at high pressure into the superfici
This causes the superficial veins to become conges... and
dilate leading to the appearance of varicose veins close to the
surface of the skin.

Varicose veins are described usually as knot-like, twisting en-
largements of the veins usually just below the skin of the legs.
Varicose means dilated or expanded and this is caused by the
breakdown of valves which are found at regular intervals in the
veins.

These varicose veins are no longer able to function properly
and other normal veins have taken over for them.

To get matters in perspective, the bigger, deep veins in the
leg carry 90% of the blood to the heart. These veins do not
become varicose because the muscle layers which surround
them protect the walls of these veins. The surface or superficial
veins only carry 10% of the blood returning to the heart. These
surface veins are the only ones which become varicose.

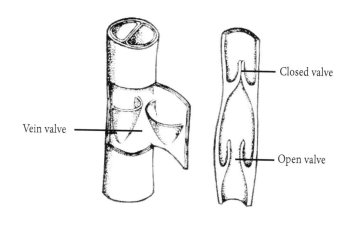

Vein valve

Closed valve

Open valve

Varicose Veins

Varicose veins are a very common condition, affecting 50% of the population in developed countries to some degree. The good news however is that for at least two-thirds of the diagnosed varicose vein population, the condition is medically insignificant, meaning these people can live with the problem with no adverse health effects.

For the remaining one-third, varicose veins do present a significant medical problem, giving rise to physical symptoms of heaviness and aching of limbs, sometimes accompanied by cramps and swollen ankles.

Varicose veins can be a progressive condition. Once a vein has started to dilate, its walls become weak and its valves dysfunction making the situation worse.

Treatment can be as simple as removing tight shoes, elevating feet periodically, walking about frequently instead of constantly standing and wearing compression stockings. More serious cases could involve medical or surgical treatment.

Varicose veins are, of course, very noticeable on the inner side of the leg, knee and thigh.

CVI (Chronic Venous Insufficiency)

This is the next step in the venous disease process that can lead to venous leg ulcers.

As you can see from the previous pie chart, venous diseases are made up mostly of varicose vein problems. Chronic Venous Insufficiency, or CVI, can then develop in a smaller percentage of the population with an unfortunate minority actually developing a venous leg ulcer.

How do you know you have CVI?

There can be many causes contributing to CVI but for the most part it is the continuation of the worsening of the varicose vein problem.

The demise of the valves means that "high pressure" blood during the contraction phase of the muscle pumping blood from the deep veins to the superficial veins (nearer the skin) creates pressures that the smaller superficial veins just cannot tolerate. This means extensive damage can be done to the delicate tissues including capillaries (tiny blood vessels) and other tissues. The bottom line of this damaging process is that harmony no longer exists in the smooth transition of fluid and oxygen exchanges between the small blood vessels (capillaries) in the body tissues.

The most significant damaging aspect of this process is the blood "pooling" in the lower leg venous system. Swelling or edema of the tissues occur which means more fluid and substances accumulate resulting in less oxygen for the tissues. This lack of oxygen contributes to the damaging of tissues, the first step towards the formation of a leg ulcer.

In some ways it would make more sense to call the venous problem VENOUS HYPERTENSION instead of CVI, because just like high blood pressure (or hypertension) the swelling of the legs is due to HIGH VENOUS BLOOD PRESSURE.

To help understanding, the following chart shows the reason for the symptoms experienced with a venous ulcer.

Symptoms Of Venous Leg Ulcers

SYMPTOM	REASON
Swelling (edema) in the legs or ankles	High venous pressure stretches vessel walls letting fluid leak out
Staining	High venous pressure stretches walls letting the red blood cells leak out
Pain when leg is down	Gravity pulls more blood down the leg
Pain relieved when leg is up	Gravity helps blood flow to the heart
Skin surface moist	Plenty of fluid in the area
Red surface	Lots of blood in the area, not moving properly
Tired, aching feeling	Too much blood in the vein causing increased pressure on the vein walls
Varicose vein appearance	Increased blood pressure in the vein causes stretching and twisting of the vein near the skin surface
Wound drainage	Leaking fluid in the area

CVI can develop over years and the end result of these processes and degradation of the skin tissues can be the development of venous leg ulcers. Often the trigger can be the patient scratching the skin of a leg which has been made eczematous (itchy) by CVI.

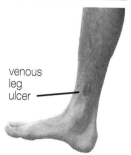

venous leg ulcer

The venous leg ulcer appearance.

The symptoms of CVI can be subtle but there is no mistaking the arrival of the venous leg ulcer, as shown above.

Often there is a strong offensive odour associated with the leg ulcer.

Usually it occurs on the inside surface of the leg just above the ankle. The shape is usually irregular and it can have a red or yellow coloring.

There is usually swelling (edema) around the lower leg area with some red or brownish staining.

One key indication that you have a venous leg ulcer is the relief of pain when the leg is elevated—when you are lying down and your legs are stretched out 6" above your heart.

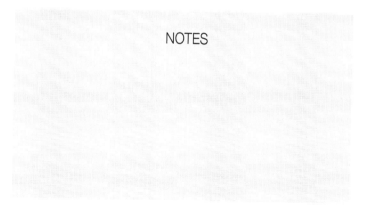

NOTES

TESTING & ASSESSING LEG ULCERS

Observation alone permits diagnosis of an existing leg ulcer. Also, the symptoms listed previously can provide those all-important warnings that you are at risk and they should be the "alarm bells" to spur you to seek help from your physician.

The physician and nurse have a range of objective ways of providing more in-depth information as to the nature of the problems. In order for you to understand the tests here are a few you may experience:

1. MEASURING BLOOD FLOW
a) Doppler Ultrasound machine

This is the size of a large pen or pencil. It is used to listen to blood flow across your skin through the aid of a gel-like substance which is used between the skin and the doppler probe (this is a sort of sophisticated microphone).

These machines have been used for many years to assess circulation problems and have been improved and refined over the years. The establishment of venous disease, its severity, the appropriateness of certain treatment and monitoring treatment are just some of the ways a doppler test can help.

Your physician or nurse may place the probe over a vein and squeeze your calf muscle to empty the vein. As they release the pressure they will listen to determine if blood is flowing back down the leg, which is what will happen if the valves in veins are not working properly.

The Doppler machine is used for one of the most important blood circulatory diagnostic tests called the ANKLE BRACHIAL PRESSURE INDEX (ABPI) which will tell your medical team how well your arteries are functioning. This is very important because it allows the physician to know how well fresh arterial (oxygenated) blood is getting to your legs and feet. With this information the medical team can decide on the appropriate treatment to heal the ulcer. More specifically your physician can determine whether or not compression therapy should be used.

The Ankle Brachial Pressure Index (ABPI) Test

All the physician or nurse uses is a blood pressure unit (sphygmomanometer) and a hand held Doppler ultrasound device. The test provides a ratio or index from two measurements which helps assess the efficiency of your blood circulation. here's the simple steps:

1. While lying down, the blood pressure is taken in both arms, this is called the Brachial (arm) pressure (B). The higher of the two systolic pressures is taken as the brachial pressure (B) for the ratio.

2. The blood pressure cuff is now placed on the leg just above the ankle. The Doppler ultrasound probe is placed at a 45-60 degree angle over the long axis of the artery.

3. The cuff is then inflated until the Doppler signal stops. Then keeping the Doppler over the artery, the cuff is slowly deflated until the Doppler signal returns. The number is recorded as the Ankle systolic pressure (A)

4. The ABPI is calculated by dividing the ankle systolic pressure (A) by the higher of the two arm (brachial) systolic pressure (B) — an example is shown below:

EXAMPLE OF A READING:
Date: February 28 2008
Brachial (Arm) pressure (B)
1 left 119   2 Right 127
Highest reading of 1&2 127 (B)
Ankle pressure 78 (A)

$$ABPI = \frac{A}{B} = \frac{78}{127} = \underline{0.614}$$

Date: _____
Brachial (Arm) pressure (B)
1 left _____   2 Right _____
Highest reading of 1&2 _____ (B)
Ankle pressure _____ (A)

$$ABPI = \frac{A}{B} = \underline{\hspace{2cm}} = \underline{\hspace{2cm}}$$

Interpretation of the ABPI
(adapted from Venous Leg Ulcer Guidelines *)

> 1.0   Normal – no evidence of arterial problems. Compression may be applied.

0.9 - 1.0   Minimal arterial problems. Compression may be applied.

0.7- <0.9   Moderately significant arterial problems. Caution should be exercised when applying compression.

0.5 - <0.7   Significant arterial problems. Extreme caution should be execised when applying compression.

<0.5   Severe arterial disease. (Patients experience pain at rest) Compression is contraindicated.

* It is worth noting that there can be false negatives or false positives due to underlying technical errors e.g. wrong Doppler angle, loose cuffs or other health problems such as diabetes or renal disease.

b) Duplex Ultrasound

Instead of listening to the blood flow after squeezing your calf, this machine produces a color coded picture of the flow of blood in your veins.

Your medical team can then see where your venous system is damaged by looking at the color patterns displayed on the screen as the blood flows through your veins. Such things as blood clots and the size of your veins can be seen.

c) Air Plethysmography

This term involves recording venous volume changes in the leg and is also used to look for blockages within the veins. Testing methods can vary but often a large blood pressure cuff is placed on the thigh and an air bag (or other sensor device) is placed below your knees.

Your nurse will then help you perform some simple maneuvers, such as sitting up, or standing on your tip-toes. If the volume of blood in your lower leg increases, this shows the venous blood is not efficiently leaving the leg.

d) Light Reflection (Photoplethysmography)

This procedure searches for reverse flow (downward flow) within your veins. It is a test meant to measure the function of the valves in your veins. An infra red light sensor is placed on your ankle and you are then asked to move your ankle ten times in order to evacuate the foot and ankle of blood. Then the sensor measures how long it takes for blood to refill the superficial (close to the surface of the leg) veins of the ankle and foot. If the refill time is too fast, this indicates the blood is flowing backwards to the superficial veins.

e) Segmental Pressure Measuring

This is just a series of blood pressure measurements taken along the leg to evaluate if a where a blockage exists. These readings may be taken high in the thigh, low in the thigh, high on the calf and on the ankle.

f) Treadmill Exercise Test

You will be asked to walk on a treadmill for a few minutes and then have your pulse and blood pressure checked afterwards. This test will tell your medical team a lot about your ability to exercise and the condition of your circulatory system.

g) Venography

Here a dye is injected into your veins and then an X-ray is taken to highlight the health of your veins.

h) Foot (Ambulatory) Venous Pressure

A small probe is inserted into the vein of your foot and measurements taken.

Venous testing is not an unpleasant experience, no anesthetic is needed and it usually takes less than one hour. It is important to avoid having coffee, tea or cigarettes at least one hour before the tests because these may affect the circulation in both your veins and arteries.

2. BLOOD ANALYSIS

Your blood can be sampled and analyzed for a whole range of tests including anemia and diabetes. The purpose is to find out if there are any underlying diseases that can interfere with healing an ulcer.

3. SWABS OF THE ULCER

These can be taken to test for infection and to check which antibiotic is the right one.

4. BLOOD PRESSURE

Your blood pressure will be regularly checked; high blood pressure can contribute to a particular pattern of ulceration.

5. PHOTOGRAPHS

Sometimes a picture is taken of the wound to monitor progress.

6. DIETARY ASSESSMENT

Nutrition is a critical factor in the healing process of venous leg ulcers. As well as obtaining adequate water and calories, the patient needs vitamins A and C, protein, iron, calcium and zinc to ensure optimum healing. A complete assessment is needed to ensure a correct nutritional program. There is no question that good nutrition can help prevent complications and accelerate wound healing. Early intervention is the key. Often the dietitian or health care practitioner will recommend appropriate supplements to achieve optimum nutrition for a particular patient.

7. PATCH TESTS

These are done to avoid an allergic reaction to a dressing, an antibiotic or topical medication. The medical team may test by placing the substances to be investigated on your back and leaving them for 48 hours, then examining and re-examining them after 72 hours.

Any allergic reactions by the body to treatment would of course have an adverse effect on healing, especially as these substances can be applied to the body for longer than a week at a time.

8. MONITORING ULCERS

Aside from these tests your medical team will keep records to monitor progress of the leg ulcer. By doing this, the progress of the ulcer can be evaluated and appropriate changes in treatment made to speed up healing. This has to be done as objectively as possible, using measuring devices. A simple way is to measure with a ruler the maximum and minimum widths. Or the outline of the ulcer can be traced on transparent material. Here are some of the guidelines the medical team uses to document and subsequently monitor the ulcer:

Location	Edge characteristics
The history - duration	Size - (depth, length and breadth)
Condition of surrounding skin	Amount of staining visible
Appearance of wound bed	Swelling
Nature of wound drainage	Amount/type of odour
Amount of pain/discomfort	Previous ulceration

In conclusion, the leg ulcer assessment is a detailed activity requiring a large amount of information so that appropriate treatment decisions can be made.

NOTES

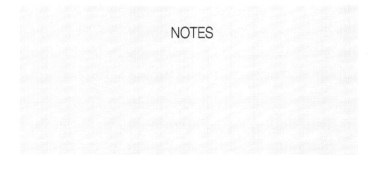

VISITING YOUR PHYSICIAN

One of the dangers of health professionals being immersed in the descriptive and objective assessment of venous leg ulcer is that they may forget about the actual "whole" patient.

Attached to that leg ulcer is a person with feelings, a medical history, a lifestyle, a family, eating habits, social commitments and so on. So although the medical team will assess the skin, the blood circulation, the limb and the actual ulcer, the "whole" patient has to be evaluated.

The physician will also assess nutrition, social circumstances, medical history, contributing risk factors, associated diseases, build, height and weight, amongst other factors.

He or she is likely to want to know the following: Do you smoke? Do you have allergies? How much do you exercise each week? What diseases have you experienced? Has your weight fluctuated? How mobile are you? Are you depressed? Do you have help at home? Do you consider yourself overweight? How would you describe your living environment? And so on. These and many other questions can be very important in the development of your treatment plan.

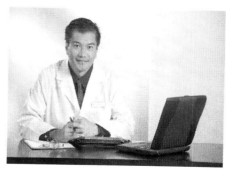

Be prepared to answer honestly. It can help if you prepare before your first visit. Think about the above questions so that you are prepared.

One of the biggest factors in successful treatment is a positive attitude and a willingness to co-operate with the treatment. Psychological support is essential for the patient together with plenty of explanations as to what is going on in treatment, expectations of progress and so on.

Your First Step

The family physician is often regarded as the "gatekeeper" for medical diagnosis and subsequent management of ill health. This is certainly true for assessing leg ulcers and then referring the patient for more specialized help. On average a family physician will see six leg ulcer patients each month. Often the family physician will start treatment immediately, usually prescribing stockings or bandaging.

So this should be your first step: **see your family physician.**

If you have not been to your physician for a while, here are a few tips to make the encounter as productive as possible:

• When you phone for an appointment let the nurse or receptionist know the reason for your consultation. If you have a leg ulcer, the quicker you arrange the appointment, the quicker it will probably heal.

• Write down questions you want to ask beforehand.

• Be aware and remind yourself of your past medical history and the history of your immediate family (heredity can give the physician many clues).

- Know exactly what medications you are taking. This is important information.

- Jot down all the symptoms you have had lately with regard to the leg ulcer and anything else that may be relevant. When you are in the physician's office you can sometimes forget.

A few tips

Answer all the physician's questions honestly. For example, if you smoke, don't hide the fact from your doctor. The medical team is there to help you, not to pass judgement.

Be assertive, not passive. Ask questions until you are sure you fully understand.

Do not accept that experiencing pain in unavoidable. Be sure to mention to your physician the pain you are experiencing and seek treatment to alleviate this pain. Experiencing pain can be debilitating for you and slow down the healing process.

Finally, try to get an assessment of how long it will take to heal the leg ulcer. There is nothing worse than false expectations; you need to know in order to adapt and plan your life accordingly.

At the end of one or two visits you should fully understand the diagnosis and what has caused the problem. There may be additional problems associated with your leg ulcer. You may well have been referred to a specialist or a retailer for tests, further assessments or for the fitting of products.

> **KEY POINTS**
>
> Prepare before your consultation, write down questions, concerns etc.
>
> Make sure you find out realistic expectations for healing time.
>
> Do not ignore any pain you experience; bring it up with your physician.

VISITING YOUR FAMILY PHYSICIAN

Questions I should ask

Medicines I am taking

Symptoms or discomfort to discuss

THE RISK FACTORS

We now understand the way leg ulcers develop from varicose veins and chronic venous insufficiency—the breakdown of valves in the veins and the swelling of tissues and so on.

However, why this happens with certain individuals and not with others is more difficult to pinpoint. A brief overview is listed below; some factors you can do nothing about, while others you can control.

Many of these risk factors are just suggestive and not conclusive and there is no way of being absolutely certain they are relevant to you.

RISKS YOU CAN CONTROL

Occupations

If you have a job which requires long periods of standing without muscular exertion (for example, hairdressers, pharmacists, factory workers, teachers, nurses, shop assistants, flight attendants etc.) then you could be at risk of developing varicose veins.

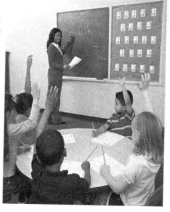

The theory is that the standing position places increased pressure on the walls and valves of the veins in the legs. Also, without subsequent muscular contractions of the legs there is little pumping action of the blood to push blood from the veins upwards.

Clearly, you can rectify this situation by moving your legs, sitting when appropriate, taking exercise breaks or even changing jobs if possible.

Restrictive clothing

Tight clothing could have an adverse effect on blood circulation. As this is one factor that can be dealt with fairly easily, it would make sense to avoid restrictive clothing. Crossing your legs could also have the same adverse effect so avoid this, too.

Pregnancy

Although the formation of varicose veins associated with pregnancy may be temporary, it has been shown the risk of developing varicose veins doubles with two or more pregnancies. In fact, it's estimated that up to 40% of all pregnant women develop varicose veins.

The reason for becoming more susceptible to varicose veins is due to an increase in certain hormone production resulting in the relaxation of vein walls, making them stretch out, and the greater blood flow to and from the womb, along with the size and weight of the expanding tummy puts additional pressure on the veins of your leg.

The major preventive actions you can take are ensuring you get plenty of rest, elevating the feet above the heart and the use of compression stockings which are explained later on in the booklet.

Trauma or injury

A knock or injury to the leg or ankle can damage the skin and contribute to an ulcer developing if you are already vulnerable to leg ulcers through venous disease.

Try making your surroundings safe so that you do not bang into objects in your home or fall because of slippery mats or protruding objects. Remember: An ounce of prevention is worth a pound of "sore".

Overweight

There have been studies to suggest that there is a link between being overweight (more specifically, being obese) and developing varicose veins. More weight puts above-average pressure on the ankle joints, makes the heart work faster and contribute to high blood pressure. Also being overweight means you have more blood and therefore the blood may "pool" in the lower legs.

The effect of excess weight is unique to each individual and your medical team needs to evaluate this factor carefully keeping in mind your medical history, body shape and other factors. Reducing weight should be done sensibly in consultation with your medical team. Do not try dramatic diets that promise huge weight losses in a short time. Weight loss must be achieved gradually in conjunction with lifestyle changes and the adoption of new positive habits that are solidified over time.

Sedentary lifestyle

Reduced physical activity has long been associated with venous disease. Remember the calf muscle is responsible for the pump function that pushes up venous blood from the legs to the heart. Obviously, if these muscles are not used, the venous blood is going to collect or pool in the legs and venous pressure will increase in the legs.

The message here is "use those calf muscles". If you do not walk much, just moving your feet upwards can help.

Smoking cigarettes

As with so many illnesses, smoking cigarettes can worsen the condition. The role smoking plays in venous leg ulcers and venous disease is that of damaging your blood circulatory system. Smoking narrows arteries, reduces oxygen within the blood vessels making your skin unhealthy and if you have a leg ulcer it slows down the healing process because less oxygen and healing nutrients are getting to the damaged skin.

Your physician or nurse can help in many ways through counseling or medical treatment. There are nicotine substitute products that can lessen the withdrawal symptoms of quitting.

Direct heat to your leg

Avoid strong, direct heat from a lamp or an electric heater, jaccuzzi or very hot baths. Although it may feel good in the short term, this type of heat can further damage your skin or aggravate an existing leg ulcer.

Skin care

The skin is the part of the body that breaks down in a venous leg ulcer so it makes sense to try and keep it as healthy as possible so that it can defend itself against the venous blood circulation problems. The main objectives of skin care are to:

a) Maintain soft, supple, clean and healthy skin
b) Prevent irritation

Your health care professionals can advise you on how to achieve these goals. There are special skin care products that can help.

Adherence to prevention or treatment

This is a major risk factor in the prevention and healing of leg ulcers!

The physician and nurse see you only a small percentage of the time. The rest of the time you have to adhere to the treatment, keep active to help circulation, avoid injury, wear correct stockings properly, eat right, and so on.

The onus is truly with the patient, caregiver, health care worker to all work together to eliminate these risks. With cooperation, an existing ulcer can be healed more quickly or, better still, a venous ulcer can actually be prevented.

As you can see there is a lot you can do to help yourself. You must not underestimate your role in achieving a successful health outcome

RISKS YOU CANNOT CONTROL

Now for the bad news: many people are predisposed to developing venous disease and subsequent venous leg ulcers, simply by virtue of who they are and their stage of life. Here are a few of the uncontrollable factors:

Heredity

One study found that the risk of developing venous disease was doubled for people with a relative with the condition. Certainly the thickness of vein walls and the number and position of vein valves varies greatly among individuals. There is a tendency to inherit weak vein walls and a low number of venous valves from

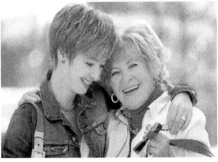

family members.

There are further sug-
gestions that the inher-
ited factor could be an
enzyme or chemical
defect responsible for
weakening the muscles
of the vein walls and al-
tering certain tissues.

Clearly if you know of direct family members who suffer from
varicose veins or venous disease, then you should take preventive action to protect yourself physically from further deteriora-
tion of the venous system.

Deep vein thrombosis (DVT)

This is a medical condition that can contribute to varicose
veins and venous leg ulceration but it is difficult to diagnose and
its true prevalence is difficult to estimate.

Deep vein thrombosis is a blood clot which has developed
within the large, deep veins of the leg.

Long periods of bed rest or periods of bed rest after a surgical
operation can contribute to the development of the problem.
One study showed DVT to have developed in 29% of over 1000
patients who had just had a surgical operation. Other factors
which can contribute to the development of DVT include the
oral contraceptive pill, obesity and pregnancy.

Aging

As venous disease is a progressive, time-driven, destructive
process, it is common sense to expect the varicose veins and
associated venous disease to worsen as time passes. The skin
thins out with age and of course that means less protection and
more vulnerability to skin damage, either through injury or the

venous disease process.

Simply looking after yourself better and taking the preventive measures we will describe later on can compensate for aging problems.

KEY POINTS

There are risks you can control.

Physical exercise, stopping smoking and adherence to treatment or prevention are the top three actions anyone can take.

RISKS I SHOULD BE CONCERNED ABOUT

TREATMENT OF VENOUS LEG ULCERS

Your resources

The treatment of venous leg ulcers can be undertaken by a wide variety of practitioners in a wide variety of settings. You may be initially seen in one setting and find your treatment occurs at another. For example, you might first go to your family physician who may assess the ulcer and send you to a vascular surgeon. After some tests, the surgeon may recommend you receive treatment at a wound healing center attached to the hospital or have a home care nurse visit you at home. The following is a list of some of the professionals and places you may come across:

Health care professionals	Places you may be treated
Family Physician	Doctor's office
Podiatrist	Podiatrist office
Home Care Nurse	Hospital
Physical Therapist	Out Patient clinic.
Vascular Surgeon	Wound Care center
Vascular Nurse	Vascular Clinic
Plastic Surgeon	Home (visit by home care nurse)
Dermatologist	Specialist's office
Gerontologist	Long term care facility
Wound Specialist Nurse	Nursing Home.
Health Worker	
Nurse Practitioner/Physician Assistant	

Purchase of supplies

Home care retailer

Drug store / pharmacy

Medical supplies retailer

Mail order catalogue

Hospital shop

Direct from medical professional

Your medical team can tell you what is covered and what is not and can give you some advice on how to acquire and pay for supplies and services.

> **KEY POINTS**
>
> Treatment is usually a team effort from various people who want to help you.
>
> Keep an open dialogue with all your contacts. You can always learn something new that may help you.

TREATMENT OPTIONS

Over the years there have been many different treatments for venous leg ulcers. Recent medical evidence has shown some new variations on old treatments that may dramatically improve the healing of your ulcer and further avoid recurrence. In the light of what you have learned from this booklet, these treatments should make sense to you.

We cannot emphasize enough that you are the key player in the treatment plan - adhering to treatment instructions and focusing on prevention tips can make the healing process much, much faster.

Treatment focuses on four separate but interrelated categories: A) Chronic Venous Insufficiency -the underlying condition; B) Wound Care -the ulcer surface; C) Surrounding Skin Care, and D) Treatment of pain associated with the ulcer. We'll look at the options for each category:

A. COMPRESSION

The swelling (edema) is primarily caused by high venous pressure. High blood pressure in your veins, is also known as venous hypertension.

1. Compression bandaging

It is widely recognized and documented that venous leg ulcers require compression of the lower leg to heal effectively. Compression reduces the swelling (edema) in the lower leg, reduces pain and helps the blood to move out of the leg back to the heart.

Compression provides a counter force to venous hypertension and forces small blood vessels to shrink back to normal so that fluid and cells no longer leak out of the blood vessels and oxygen and nutrients can be transported in the normal fashion.

Even old leg ulcers that have not responded to other treatments will be helped by properly applied compression systems. Compression systems may also contribute to healing of leg ulcers that have not responded to other forms of treatments. Compression is required to aid the restoration of normal blood flow to the lower leg. Before healing can occur, it is necessary to reduce the swelling (edema) in the leg.

There are two types of compression used: rigid bandages (short stretch), have little stretching capacity. While Elastic bandages (long stretch) are less rigid and contain more stretching capacity.

Rigid (inelastic) compression

Unna's Boot

This most common form of treatment has been around for over 100 years. It was developed by a doctor named Unna and is called the Unna's Boot. With this therapy, a moist bandage is wrapped around the lower leg and covered with another bandage to keep the moist bandage protected from soiling. The moist bandage usually contains a zinc oxide base and may contain other ingredients to assist in providing moisture and reduce skin irritation. The zinc oxide bandage is wrapped around the lower leg from the base of the toes to just below the knee forming a rigid tube.

This creates pressure which helps push blood up the leg and back to the heart. The Unna's Boot helps keep swelling (edema) down which helps oxygen and nutrients within the blood get to the ulcer and aid in the healing process.

There are all kinds of combinations of dressings and bandages used together that are called "Unna's Boots" but most of them share the moist zinc oxide paste bandages the first layer and they are usually applied for a full week at a time.

It is important to remember that the Unna's Boot works best when combined with exercise such as walking. You will want to stay active and work your muscle pump and not expect the bandage to do all the work.

Other types of inelastic (rigid) compression

Other types of bandages can be used to help take advantage of your muscle pump. Rigid (short stretch) bandages are specifically designed to contain little stretch and provide a high resistance. You can recognize them by the fact that they are not stretchy when you put them on. They are like the paste bandages previously discussed but without the paste.

They will also be applied around the leg from the base of the toe to just below the knee.

This type of bandaging may be taken off at night or when bathing. It is important to put the bandage on first thing in the morning to keep the swelling down. Remember that swelling is your enemy so keep these products on whenever you are standing.

Another form of rigid compression is a device with many straps that wrap around the leg and are tightly fastened with velcro closures. Again, if you remove it at night or when bathing or showering, make sure you put it back on first thing in the morning.

Elastic Compression

You can recognize elastic bandages by the way they stretch and pull back when you release them. Elastic bandages also supply pressure to your leg when applied. They work with your muscle pumps and provide constant compression when exercising. They are designed to provide an external counter pressure to your leg that works to reduce the effect of the high venous pressure that led to your ulcer.

There are two main types of elastic bandages to treat venous ulcers. The first type is moderate compression elastic and the second type is high compression elastic bandages.

Elastic bandages may also be used in the new multi – layered compression systems.

High compression elastic bandages feel strong when you stretch them and may have little squares or indicators that allow you to determine when you have stretched them properly.

They are often applied by themselves over a padding bandage. You may be required to remove your compression bandage at night and put it on again first thing in the morning. Some bandaging systems may be worn for up to a full week. A health care professional should direct you on how long to wear the compression bandaging systems.

Moderate compression bandages do not feel as strong when you pull them on and usually don't supply enough compression when used alone. They are often used as part of a multi – layer compression system.This allows continued compression even after the swelling subsides.

Several multi layer compression systems are available that take advantage of the different properties of individual layers. They may vary in layers; some contain three while others contain four layers. Most are left on for up to a week to keep your leg under contiuous compression.

You may use a multi layer system if you are not comfortable applying your own bandage everyday or if your medical team wants to make certain your leg is always under control. Recent studies have shown that, in general, multi layer systems perform best over single wraps and elastic compression systems perform better than inelastic systems.

You may think that because of all the pressure they put on your leg, compression bandages will be uncomfortable. In fact most people find they are more comfortable and have less pain when their leg is under compression. By providing a counter pressure to your venous hypertension, they keep swelling down, improve the blood flow to your leg and reduce the damage and pain caused by the stretching of your blood vessels. Studies have shown that people take fewer pain relievers when they are using good compression products. In the light of all this positive evidence they are worth giving a try -you may be pleasantly surprised

A health care professional will assess the needs of each individual; take critical measurements such as limb radius and the amount of swelling. Once the assessment is complete the bandage will then be applied to the appropriate pressure required.

Successful outcome using compression therapy depends on the initial application of the bandage and patient cooperation. It is important for the patient to receive education and follow up visits once therapy is initiated.

There are many decisions to be made by the health care professional such as: the distribution of pressure, the duration of pressure, the types of bandage and the number of bandages to be applied.

The people who fit these bandages are extremely well trained but it is really important for you to voice your concerns or ask for it to be explained again if you do not understand something.

Key principles of compression bandaging:

1. Compression bandaging should not be used if there is arterial disease and leg ulcers associated with diabetes. More damage can occur in the ulcer or within the blood circulation system.

2. There should be graduated compression—greatest at the ankle while decreasing as it is applied up the leg. Compression is measured in millimeters (mm) of mercury (Hg). Although everyone's needs are different, the general rule, is 32 – 42 mm Hg at the ankle (if tolerated) and ending with 12 – 17 mmHg below the knee.

3. Overly tight bandaging should be avoided. This may cause too much constiction resulting in persistent pain.

4. Compression to the ulcerated area alone is ineffective.

5. The bandage must be applied from the toe to the knee - molding around the ankle, up to the level just below the knee.

6. The bandage must not be applied directly to the ulcer or to skin which is damaged or inflamed. A dressing or a paste bandage must act as a buffer.

7. After healing, further compression may be necessary to prevent recurrence. At this point a compression stocking may be appropriate.

8. Patient co-operation is absolutely vital when using a compression bandage. For example, the elevation of legs just above the heart when the opportunity arises further helps the compression treatment. Also complete explanations from the health care professional on usage, warning signs is critical.

2. Compression hosiery (stockings)

Therapeutic Stockings are similar in treatment principles to compression bandaging. There are some important differences between these two types of therapy. For example, one important feature of compression bandaging is the unique form fitting, when applied. Compression Hosiery works collaboratively with the calf muscles for a dual effect, which assists the venous valves to close. The weave and the fabric of each stocking creates slight recoil tension, thereby exerting a constant, gently pressure on the limb. Hence, the action of the stocking pushes inwards onto the limb, while the calf muscles push outwards. The benefit of this dual effect, assists the venous valves to close and sufficiently return blood and fluids back to the heart. additionally, the stocking counteracts the high pressures in your leg thus preventing further fluid build up. Pain and swelling are reduced, comfort is improved, while further ulcer development is avoided.

There is a wide range of compression hosiery available. Different brands, different shapes, different sizes and different styles. There are knee high, thigh high, and full pantyhose styles. It is important to choose the appropriate compression in order to achieve consistent therapeutic benefit.

The Four Categories of Compression Hosiery

1) Support Wear:
Contains a very mild compression of 8-5 mmHg
- Tired aching legs
- Mild swelling
- prevention for people who are required to stand, or sit in one position for long periods of time.

2) Medical Leg Wear:

Is available in compressions from 15-50 mmHg
- Management and prevention of venous leg ulcer minor to severe varicosities
- Minor to severe edema
- Post-surgery and sclerotherapy
- Pregnancy related edema and varicosities
- Lymphatic edema
- Management of Chronic Venous Insufficiency

3) Custom Wear:

Is available in compression of 15-90 mmHg
- Patients with abnormal limb shapes
- Patients who need an unlimited size range
- Patients who need specific garment options to improve compliance and fit (i.e. zippers reinforcements, linings, contracture seams, ostomy openings, abdominal panels)
- patients who need long-term management of lyphedema, or vascular edema

4) Ulcer Care:

Contains a compression of 40 mmHg
- Stocking designed specifically for use with venous ulcerations
- Two parts system providing a total pressure of 40+ mmHg
- Liner holds dressing in place, is easy to don and is worn 24 hrs/day, facilitates donning of Outer stocking
- This stocking is used until the ulceration heals
- Outer stocking has zipper to facilitate donning and is worn during ambulation over the white liner
- Open toe stocking

Unfortunately, venous hypertension which caused your leg ulcer does not go away. Once your ulcer has healed, you will need to wear these stockings as a preventive measure in order to keep compression on the leg whenever you are not lyng down.

As with a compression bandage, the correct fitting of the stocking by a professional is vital for a successful health outcome.

Ideally the leg should be measured at the beginning of the day to minimize the effect of swelling. If this is not possible then the patient must rest for a while with legs elevated just before measurement. Measurements should be made with the patient's feet flat on the ground and should be taken for both legs as variances may occur and different sizes for each leg may be necessary.

Your measurements:

Circumference of the narrowest part
of the ankle _____

Circumference at the widest part of the calf_____

Length of the leg from the heel to just below the knee
(for knee length) _____

Length of the leg from the heel to the groin
(for full size) _____

Foot length_____

A follow-up appointment is usually arranged after the hosiery has been fitted to ensure that the hosiery is being used properly. Regular review may be required to check for any problems.

Ideally, new hosiery should be re-ordered every four to six months.

Do not buy more than one pair on the first time to make sure that your choice is right for your needs.

Finally, to eliminate two common misconceptions: a) compression stockings **DO NOT** damage blood circulation; on the contrary they assist venous circulation in the legs and: b) compression stockings **DO NOT** weaken the muscles in the leg. Walking will provide the exercise to maintain muscle tone.

The main purpose of compression hosiery is to prevent leg ulcers and avoid recurrence. It is also used to reduce venous hypertension on a sustained long term basis.

Again, it is critical that people know how to apply their compression hosiery. See the self help tips on compression hosiery to be sure you are doing everything correctly.

Here are the instructions for wearing stockings:

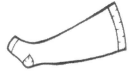

1. Your stocking.

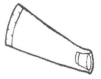

2. turn stocking inside out up to heel.

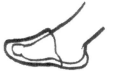

3. Place your slipper over your foot.

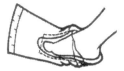

4. Pull foot of stocking over your foot.

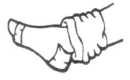

5. Slowly ease stocking up over heel and ankle.

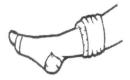

6. Gently ease the rest of the stocking a bit at a time up the leg

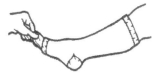

7. Pull slipper liner through the opening of the toes.

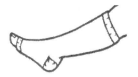

8. if this is a knee length stocking, the top should go no further than the crease behind your knee.

There should be no creases or wrinkles. The stocking should fit smoothly along the leg.

STOCKING DIARY RECORD

Name: _____ Height: _____ Foot Size: _____

DATE	ANKLE CIRCUM	CALF CIRCUM	THIGH CIRCUM	HIP CIRCUM	WEIGHT	STOCKING BRAND	STOCKING SIZE	COLOR

B. WOUND CARE - the ulcer surface

Though maintaining proper compression is the key to healing your venous leg ulcer you will also need to take care of the actual wound as it heals. Nature sets a healing time for each type of wound but that healing will only occur if there are favorable conditions for the ulcer to heal. Wounds must be kept clean, (free from debris and infection), warm (not hot), protected from the outside environment and allowed to stay moist (not wet).

Your nurse or health worker has been trained to create these favorable conditions and of course the use of dressings for a particular ulcer is a critical factor in the healing process.

For your information these are the steps that can be taken in professional physical aspects of ulcer care:

Cleansing

Most of the time your medical team will rinse the ulcer surface with a simple salt (saline) solution. This will be formulated to be as close as possible to the normal salt concentration in your body fluids. Rinsing the wound removes any dirt or dressing material that may have accumulated. It also washes out excess fluid (wound exudate) and germs. Healing ulcers after cleansing have a nice red shiny appearance and the medical team now has an ideal opportunity to assess the wound's progress from the previous treatment.

During the first few visits it may be necessary to be a little more aggressive at cleansing. The wound may have accumulated some yellow or black material or may have more germs than the medical team would like. You must appreciate all leg ulcers have some contamination and this does not appear to slow the healing process.

An important principle in cleansing the ulcer surface is not to damage newly formed healing cells. The frequency and appropriateness of cleansing is the decision of the health care professional but certainly on the first visit they will want to get you off to the best possible start.

Other cleansing activities:

Debridement: This is the term used for the physical removal of any blood clots, scabs or dry crust on the ulcer through mechanical, chemical or surgical means. This removal of dead tissue can speed up the healing process.

Mechanical debridement can be simple wiping the wound with a gauze sponge or leaving a wet gauze in the wound until it dries and picks up the debris.

Chemical debridement can be achieved using certain solutions or biological solutions called enzymes to dissolve the unwanted material from the ulcer surface.

Surgical debridement can simply be the picking out bits of damaged tissue using tweezers or cutting bebris out with a scalpel.

For most people with venous leg ulcers, aggressive debriding is not necessary as venous leg ulcers are the "healthiest" of the leg ulcer family and tend not to accumulate ulcer surface debris. Simple cleansing or effective dressings that help clean (autolytic debriding) the wound are usually quite sufficient.

Hydrotherapy is a cleansing technique whereby rushing water treats the wound. You would sit with your lower leg in a water tank while a jet of water rushes over the wound to rinse out any contaminants. After a few treatments of hydrotherapy and good compression therapy the need for hydrotherapy should be drastically reduced.

Finally **antibiotics or antimicrobials** may be used to clear up an infection within the ulcer. You may have a topical antibiotic applied to the ulcer surface and or you may take an antibiotic by mouth. Also the cleansing solution may be modified to include one with an antimicrobial agent included until the infection is cleared up. Your medical team may or may not stop other treatments.

Venous leg ulcers are not normally a high risk for infection, however, infection is possible with any wound and you will want to know the signs and report them to your medical team if they occur. These signs include: increased redness around the ulcer, the ulcer area seems hot to touch and the area around the ulcer may show additional swelling other than the general swelling of the leg.

Surgical procedures

If your ulcer is larger than average or not healing as quickly as expected, the medical team may suggest speeding things up with a skin graft of which your surgeon will explain the advantages of the different types.

The two most commonly used are:

a) *Partial thickness graft.* - as the name suggests, the surgeon uses a special knife (dermatome) to take a very thin slice of skin from your upper leg or back (donor site) that will be used to cover your ulcer. As the slice is very thin the donor site will heal quickly. After placing the skin over your ulcer the area is covered with a dressing and inspected every few days to make sure the graft ' takes'

b) *Pinch graft* — instead of completely covering the ulcer with skin your team may decide to take small pinches of skin from your thigh and place them in your leg ulcer. These pinch grafts form little 'islands' of healthy skin that grow out toward each other until your ulcer is completely covered.

Artificial skin substitutes are another alternative which is developing momentum because of the reduced likelihood of rejection of the products. You will benefit of course from less discomfort from not having skin taken from your body but more important there appears to be a much quicker healing time with a brand new product—a bilayered Human Skin Equivalent (HSE) which seems to be revolutionizing venous leg ulcer treatment.

Your physician simply grafts a strip over the ulcer rather like a large band - aid -only this band - aid is living. Because it is so similar to human skin, it rapidly adheres to the exposed ulcer and stimulates healing. Eventually the strip is replaced by the patient's own skin. This is only just being made available and its unique medical classification can create problems in billing procedures.

Finally a vascular or plastic surgeon can contribute to the healing process by surgically altering the skin and tissue around the ulcer and thereby provide a more favorable structure conducive to healing. This is a marginal surgical approach but can be very beneficial.

DRUG THERAPY

Other than antibiotics there are few drugs that can improve the healing of your venous leg ulcer. You may have been prescribed analgesic medication to reduce the pain you may feel; however you can expect the need for analgesics will decrease as your ulcer gets better.

There are some medications that increase the ability of oxygen carrying red blood cells to reach the wound and these may be helpful for some patients.

A new class of drugs called "growth factors" has recently become available and these may be indicated if your venous ulcer is slow to heal. The drug's generic category is PDGF

-Platelet- Derived Growth Factor and simply mimics the body's natural 'healing' platelet activities. The drug is recombinant (not derived from blood) and is available by prescription.

DRESSINGS

The vast majority of venous leg ulcers require nothing more than good compression to manage the underlying high venous pressure and appropriate dressings to protect and manage the wound surface while the ulcer is healing. As the ulcer heals it gets smaller, more shallow (superficial) and the type and amount of moisture it produces changes. Each time your wound is assessed the team may decide to either stay with the current dressing or to change to one more appropriate to the condition of the wound at that time.

As the venous leg ulcer is only a symptom of the underlying problem with venous pressure, your team may use something quite simple as a wound contact layer. Early in the course of treatment your wound may be putting out a lot of fluid (exudate) trying to clean itself out. At this point the team may choose a dressing that will absorb a lot of fluids between changes and help the wound to clean itself. Later your wound will be a shiny red color with very little drainage (exudate) so they can use a dressing designed to absorb less fluid and keep the wound protected, warm and moist. You may be quite surprised at the number of dressings available to your medical team, here's a few general categories:

1. **Wound Contact layer-** As the name suggests, are simple dressings designed to go into the wound and isolate it from other dressings or bandages that will placed over the

wound. The wound contact layer will be very thin and allow any excess fluid (exudate) produced by your ulcer to pass through to other dressings or absorbent bandages. The wound contact layer may be dry or coated to ensure nothing sticks to your wound as it heals, many dressings have the wound contact layer built right in so you may not notice one in your dressing mix.

2. **High Absorption dressings** - when your wound is producing a lot of fluid (exudate) it may a little help to avoid becoming too wet. Think about what happens to your skin if you spend too much time in a warm bath. The skin softens and swells as it absorbs more and more water. The result is called skin maceration and the fluid produced by your wound can lead to the same result if not wicked away from your skin. Some of the material that can handle a lot of fluid include :

Foam, Fibers (woven into a pad like a gauze pad), Alginates (absorbent pads derived from seaweed), Hydrocolloid sheets (a brown thick paste of cellulose), covered pouches or pads), hydrofibers (highly absorbent processed fibers) and Absorptive / padding bandages (looks like cast padding and worn under compression bandages)

3. **Low absorbent dressings** - are also made from a wide variety of appropriate materials to keep just the right amount of moisture over your ulcer, such materials include: thin foams, thin hydrocolloids, hydrogels (clear gel pads or pastes) and transparent films (looks like Saran Wrap)

All these materials mentioned can be used in various combinations to produce composite dressings.

Dressings may have an adhesive that glues them to the skin around the ulcer or may have no adhesive and rely on the compression bandage to hold them in place.

Selecting the most appropriate dressing takes into consideration a wide range of factors such as whether the goal of treatment is healing or maintenance, the amount of exudates or drainage (this determines the right absorbency qualities for the dressing), the nature of the wound bed, patient comfort and costs.

There are other more objective systematic ways of listing the various dressing types available but this description is adequate for the purposes of this book to provide understanding. The judgement skills of the medical profession will determine the appropriate dressing options for a particular patient.

Remember the leg ulcer is only a symptom of the underlying high venous pressure in the leg which causes the ulcer. Dressings only manage the symptom (the ulcer) and you will always need your compression bandage or stockings during and after ulcer healing.

Dressings will help you be more comfortable and reduce the need to change your bandages but it is always the compression that heals the wound and prevents it from coming back.

Changing a dressing

More often than not your caregiver will usually change a dressing but it's useful to be aware of the basic guidelines - you may write in any special instructions:

1. Remove all hand jewelry.

2. Wash your hands thoroughly.

3. Put on sterile gloves and check to be sure there are no breaks in the glove material. If there are then discard the gloves and start again.

4. Remove the tape around the dressing carefully from the person's skin

5. Gently remove the old dressing but don't touch any of it that touched the actual ulcer.

6. Fold the edges together, place in a disposable bag and close the bag tightly.

7. Remove your gloves and put on a fresh pair.

8. Clean and irrigate the wound and surrounding skin following the instructions from your medical team

Instructions: ──────────────────────────────

───

9. Pat dry the skin around the ulcer.

10. Apply the new dressing in accordance with your clinician and manufacturer's instructions

Other instructions: ──────────────────────

───

───

NAME OF DRESSING(S) ──────────────────

───

───

OTHER TREATMENTS
Negative Pressure Wound Therapy (NPWT)
This innovative and well proven system uses negative pressure on a wound to help promote healing through multiple mechanisms of action.

UV irradiation, UVI is a form of light therapy where a special frequency of light is shone on the ulcer for a certain period of time each week.

Hyperbaric oxygen Two forms of hyperbaric oxygen therapy are available.

1. You will sit or lie down in an oxygen chamber like the ones used to help divers recover from diving accidents and breathe air enriched with oxygen.

2. Your leg is placed in a mini chamber and topical oxygen will be concentrated at high pressure over your ulcer.

Electromagnetism magnets are used to create magnetic fields which can enhance the healing process through stimulation.

Compression Pumps

No matter what your treatment you may be following your team may decide you need a little extra help to reduce the swelling (edema) and speed up your healing. There are several types of leg pumps that encourage blood flow and reduce swelling.

The procedure involves putting your leg into a fabric or plastic sleeve with several pockets that can be inflated and inflated to assist your circulation. You may buy one or rent one for use at home or visit a clinic for your leg pumping session.

It is important to appreciate that while you may get benefits from the pumping session you will still need to maintain compression to protect your veins between sessions. So be certain to wear your bandages or stockings whenever you are not lying down.

Surgery - Vein valve transplantation

This is a very promising surgical procedure where the underlying cause of the disease, faulty valves within veins, can be repaired.

One technique involves taking healthy "vein valve segments" from one part of the patient and transplanting this healthy vein as close as possible to the symptomatic site - the place on the leg causing the most problems of ulceration, or chronic vein insufficiency.

In one trial, a group of 25 patients had severe CVI and ulcers, and 15 were found to have severe defective valve problems. Twelve of these patients underwent valve transplantation, all obtained complete relief of pain, their ulcers healed and they were able to walk once again.

However the general concensus at this time is that there are very few candidates for valve replacement surgery -other methods of treatment should be initially used.

C. SKIN CARE

Your medical team can advise you on the products that will help but the goals of looking after your skin, especially around your ulcer area, are:

a) Maintain soft, supple, clean and healthy skin.

b) Prevent skin irritation and subsequent damage

c) Improve circulation throughout the skin, with special attention to the most vulnerable areas.

The use of preventative skin care products provides you with enormous preventative and healing benefits for by the patient with fragile and compromised skin.

Some of the products may include:
I) a cleanser that will maintain the skin's healthy pH (the acidity level)

2) Moisturizing cream - which should be hypo allergenic -this will prevent dangerous itching of dry and delicate skin. Avoid at all costs scratching that itch!

3) Protective creams and ointments which will protect skin from wetness and soothe the skin thereby speeding up the healing process and preventing possible rashes.

Maintaining good skin condition with these products will also help avoid small breaks in the skin that could lead to ulcer formation.

Aside from your recommended skin care products to achieve these skin care goals here are some general tips. (Remember if you have an active ulcer you may be given specific advice for protective measures which must be absolutely followed)

• Ensure adequate bathing or showering to keep skin clean.

• Be sure not to spend too long in the bath and do not use very hot water (this can deplete natural moisture from the skin)

• Towel dry gently to avoid damaging the skin.

• Do not use harsh cleaning agents that can irritate the skin.

• Try to avoid perspiration.

Regularly inspect the skin for warning signs such as redness, burning sensations or pain. Consult your physician immediately if you suspect a problem.

My products and skin care procedures

Recommended products

How they should be used

D. PAIN MANAGEMENT

You must mention to your physician if you are experiencing a lot of discomfort and pain. While battling your ulcer you need to be as free from pain as possible to keep up your morale.

Conversely the onus is with the physician/nurse and also the caregivers and front line health workers to adopt an interventionist policy and ask the right questions to pinpoint the extent of the pain problem.

Quality of life research studies have consistently highlighted that pain is an overwhelming issue for patients living with a leg ulcer. It is unfortunate that sometimes patients accept the pain as the norm – "it comes with the territory". Further research has also shown that health workers and even professionals assume that venous leg ulcers are not painful.

Some aspects of treatment can alleviate some of the pain, venous leg ulcers are painful because nerve endings are exposed; a moist, occlusive dressing will protect the nerves and can reduce pain. Further the pain from engorged veins and swollen tissue in your legs can usually be reduced by compression from bandages or stockings and from elevating the legs.

In the event you need pain relief during dressing changes, a topical gel can be applied along the edge of the wound after cleaning it.

To relieve local pain associated with chronic venous leg ulcers, the non–narcotic varieties such as ibuprofen, acetaminophen usually help.

To provide some flavour and direction to this issue here are some research findings:

- Patients considered pain a normal or expected part of the experience of having a venous leg ulcer

- Patient mostly knew swelling equated to pain and reducing pain involved compression or elevation of the legs.

- Patients were frustrated with the problem of not being able to stand for long periods of time.

- Patients' most intense pain came from debridement and dressing changes and they considered these activities mostly unpleasant.

Research has also pinpointed many words used by patients to describe their pain such as: *aching, annoying burning, dull, hot, hurting, nagging, sharp, shooting, sick – in – the – stomach pain, stabbing, stinging, throbbing and uncomfortable.*

There are some excellent educational tools and products developed by manufacturers and health care professionals that can help. For example a pain scale has been developed, a dressing with an impregnated analgesic is being marketed in some countries.

It is important to be aware that the range of pain associated with venous ulcers can be varied. For example there can be pain and tenderness along an affected vein, a dull ache can be caused by edema, increased intensity of pain can be brought on by an infection, to name just a few.

Helpful pointers in pain management

a) Use a pain scale tool routinely, involve the patient, and educate the patient on the scale.

b) You have to accept pain is subjective but you also have to accept that the patient's perception of the pain is the reality. Ask questions to assess nature of the pain and obtain a dialogue, for example:
- Can you describe the pain?
- What word best describes your pain?
- Where is the pain?
- What makes the pain worse?
- Is the pain worse at night?
- What makes the pain better?
- Are dressing changes painful to you?
- What painkillers are you taking?

c) In order to prevent pain during a debridement or a dressing change it is important to plan and prepare based on your assessment of the patient's pain situation. Here are some suggestions:
- Explain the entire process to the patient.
- Consider preventative analgesia. (painkillers)
- Provide a non stressful environment, cell phones turned off, windows closed, quiet setting etc.
- Avoid prolonged exposure of the ulcer e.g. waiting for nurse to arrive.
- Decide if a family member or someone holding hands or touching will help.
- Constantly involve the patient in dialogue to check how they are feeling.
- Make sure the optimum dressing is being used.

HEALING TIME

There are several factors that will influence how quickly you can expect your leg ulcer to heal. You can control some of them while others depend upon the history and condition of your veins and the size and duration of your ulcer.

In general the smaller your ulcer when you begin treatment, the faster it will heal. This means it is important to seek medical help as soon as you suspect a problem.

Ulcers that are than 6 months old will heal more slowly than those that are treated earlier. It has been documented that even older ulcers react well to compression therapy and "wake up" and start healing.

This is probably due to compression therapy reducing swelling and helping bring fresh blood and subsequent nutrients to the area. In any case start treatment as soon a possible.

The more serious the underlying venous problem the longer you can expect for the ulcer to heal and the more aggressive treatment your treatment will be. Your medical team will advise you on what to expect from their assessment.

KEY POINTS

Compression is the "gold standard" treatment for venous leg ulcers.

Make sure you adher to all the instructions for compression therapy either for bandaging or stockings.

Remember you do not have to experience pain. Make sure you tell your physician or nurse how you feel.

It is important to have realistic expectations of healing times so that you can mentally prepare yourself.

BEST PRACTICE RECOMMENDATIONS

These recommendations are a concensus of expert opinion, applying the available evidence to the management of venous ulcers. The specifics can be somewhat technical so in "Reader's Digest" fashion we have paraphrased the information for ease of reading so that if you are a patient, caregiver or health worker you should understand and appreciate the proper process of treatment.

Recommendations

Identify & treat the cause

1. Obtain a careful patient history
2. Perform a physical assessment e.g. ABPI and other tests
3. Determine the cause(s) of the CVI (Chronic Venous Insufficiency)
4. Implement compression therapy (bandages / stockings)
5. Implement medical therapy if appropriate.
6. Consider surgical management

Address patient concerns

7. Communicate with patients, the family and caregivers to establish realistic expectations for healing and provide information for the care and management of the problems.

Establish the presence of social support system for the patient.

Provide wound care

8. Assess the wound
9. Provide local wound care

Provide organizational support

10. Consult appropriate disciplines within the medical team to address other factors such as mobility, nutrition and other illnesses.

You can do a lot not only to help heal the leg ulcer faster but to prevent one from developing.

For the patient, caregiver and health worker the next section is an important part of the booklet.

The key to healing and preventing leg ulcers is to reduce swelling (edema) in the legs and keep the blood moving to avoid congestion of blood in the legs. The following is a list of tips you can do something about.

MOST IMPORTANT SELF HELP TIPS

1. KEEP YOUR COMPRESSION BANDAGING IN PLACE

All members of the medical profession will tell you that compression by way of a bandage is the gold standard for venous leg ulcer care. You should follow the nurse's / physician's instructions conscientiously regarding how you manage your compression bandage in between visits; write out the recommendations of your physician if necessary, here are some principles:

- The bandage should be applied like a sleeve not a clamp, otherwise it can create a tourniquet effect and this can cause pain.

- The compression should be graduated - slowly decreasing as it moves up the leg.

- Follow the manufacturer instructions on maintenance, renewal, etc.

- Avoid producing a high band of compression in the calf region of the leg, a common mistake.

- If you have to reapply the bandage in the morning make sure you do it before you get up or have been lying down for at least half an hour.

The more time you spend under good compression the more time your ulcer is actively trying to repair itself. Each time you allow a little swelling to occur you must reduce it to start the healing process again. For this reason your medical team may decide on a system that stays on for a full week.

Are there some instructions you do not understand? Do you know why compression is important? Make a note of these.

2. EXERCISE

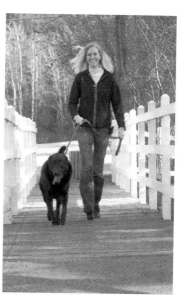

Veins do not have their own muscles to pump blood out of the leg. For this reason they rely on you using your foot and leg muscles to provide the pumping force. You do not have to join a gym and work out all day but you do need to walk and avoid standing still.

If you are not walking, lie down. If you cannot lie down then sit with your legs on a stool. If you cannot do that at least remember to exercise frequently by pushing down on your toes and raising your heels. Every bit of pumping helps speed up the healing process. Also remember exercise without compression works against you by forcing more blood into the lower leg and raising the venous pressure. Exercise only when your legs are under good compression or when you are lying down.

When traveling or otherwise out of your normal routine, do whatever exercises you can fit into the situation.

Go for walks and exercise those leg muscles in ways that work for you. Movement simply gets the blood moving. By being outside you could be stimulated, meeting people and enjoying the surroundings. Exercise makes you feel good about yourself.

If the weather is bad or you simply want to do more exercise continuously without going outside, there are exercises you can perform indoors e.g. moving your foot up and down. This exercises the calf muscles in the leg which helps pump the blood upward.

Do you need to talk to your health care practitioner about an appropriate exercise plan? Do you think you have been doing enough walking or other appropriate exercise? Make a note of these.

3. ELEVATE THE LEGS - REST PROPERLY

Just sitting down and taking a load off your feet is pleasant but you can do more:

Lie down and raise your feet higher than your heart by about six inches. This removes the problem of gravity trying to slow down the venous blood moving up your legs. Instead gravity is now working gently in your favor. Do this type of resting as frequently as possible.

Do you have somewhere at home where you can elevate your legs comfortably? If not what can you do about it?

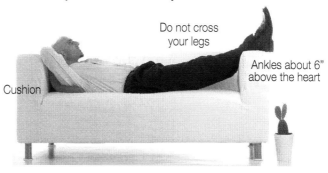

Do not cross your legs

Ankles about 6" above the heart

Cushion

4. USE COMPRESSION STOCKINGS CORRECTLY

After your leg ulcer has healed or before one develops the use of these stockings is vital to prevent swelling in the legs and therefore help prevent leg ulcers and venous problems.

Read the manufacturer's instructions and ensure proper fitting with a specialist fitter. Home care stores, pharmacies or your clinic can help you find the correct stockings.

For best results, compression stockings should be worn from dawn till dusk, all day long, every day.

They should be put on in the morning before you get out of bed. If you have left your bed without putting the stockings on, go back, lie down for a few minutes with your legs elevated and wiggle your toes to empty your veins. Remain in this position and pull on your stockings.

Your needs may change as your legs change—they may become reduced in size due to reduced swelling or may even become more muscular due to your exercise program. Keep a record of your size, and make a note of the stockings you purchased, pinpointing the date for purchasing new ones.

Use a diary record. This is important to maintain the right compression for you. The stocking will be less effective over time and as we said, your legs may have physically changed. A commonly asked question is, "Should you remove stockings if aching or tightness in the leg is experienced ?" The answer is usually, **No**. The reasons for the symptoms are due probably to a period of inactivity and a build—up of fluid in the leg. Either try to walk around or exercise the legs as shown earlier. It can also help to raise the legs as shown previously.

Compression stockings should be washed by hand in cool water with a mild soap. Wring them gently in a towel and avoid stretching them. Let them dry in the open air, away from sources of heat. And **NEVER** put them in the dryer.

73

5. ADHERENCE TO YOUR TREATMENT

Whether you are having surgery, taking medication, having stockings fitted and so on, you must make sure you fully understand what you have to do to help yourself. Furthermore, it helps to understand from your health care professional the what, why, how, when and where of your treatment so that your expectations and understanding are right.

6. ADEQUATE SKIN CARE

As well as following the tips and using the recommended products you must maintain the habit of vigilance in regular skin inspection of your lower leg. Any changes or suspect problems should be reported immediately to your medical team. Remember small fresh ulcers can heal quickly so the sooner they are detected and treated the less discomfort, bother and expense you can expect.

7. ASK FOR PAIN TREATMENT

Pain is a major quality of life issue and there is no need to accept pain as normal part of the experience of a venous ulcer. There are several options available to you that you should discuss with your medical team.

HELPFUL LIFESTYLE TIPS

1. STOP SMOKING

Good blood circulation to your ulcer is critical to successful healing. Cigarettes dramatically and destructively reduce the blood circulation to all parts of your body. Less oxygen and fewer nutrients and healing components formed by the body will get to the site of your leg ulcer.

Your physician can help you quit. There is medication available to reduce the craving of cigarettes. Many people quit after several tries. However, the one factor that seems to help the success rate of quitting is to talk the matter over with your physician. He or she can help psychologically by giving support and direction and medically by reducing the craving.

2. EAT NUTRITIOUSLY

Your body needs all the right nutrients to heal your leg ulcer. Make sure your diet is nutritious and varied, providing necessary minerals, vitamins and energy. Follow Canada's food guide. To help heal a wound plenty of water and calories are required as well as vitamins A and C, protein, iron, calcium and zinc. It is recommended to use liquid or powdered supplements and vitamins.

3. LOSE WEIGHT IF YOU NEED TO

Your medical team will advise you on this. It's common sense, though, that being overweight is hard on the joints, the heart and the veins. By reducing weight, you're putting less stress on these critical parts of the body. Also by being overweight you are carrying more than just extra fat (adipose tissue)—your body needs more blood and blood vessels to feed the fat. This means there is more blood within your body and therefore more 'pooling' can occur in the lower leg and make your venous pressure worse.

Our physician editors emphasize that it's important not to be overwhelmed at how much weight you think you must lose. The loss of just 5-10 pounds can make you feel better and improve your quality of life. Doing something simple like eliminating margarine or butter or cutting down on sweets or exercising can over the months provide you with that easy "no pain" way of losing weight.

6. SEEK SUPPORT

Family member, friends and caregivers can make all the difference in either preventing a venous leg ulcer or helping the healing process. Relieving your worries and concerns can make you feel a lot better. And don't underestimate how much people want to help. Most people like to help out --- it makes them feel good.

7. POSITIVE ATTITUDES

A chronic disease like a leg ulcer can bring on a feeling of helplessness. Seek help, discuss your feelings with a health care professional or friend, try to develop a sense of control, perhaps by completing the check list at the end of the book - everything you need to know about getting beter in included within the check list.

COMMON SENSE TIPS

1. AVOID STANDING FOR LONG PERIODS OF TIME

If your job or certain activities demand you stand without moving for long periods of time, this will usually increase swelling and hinder the healing process. You must try to be assertive and ensure that you rest properly or obtain a chair or stool. Try to move about as often as possible, exercising the legs and getting the blood moving. Sitting in cramped quarters can also be a problem which you should avoid.

2. DO NO HARM

A knock on your ulcer can set back the healing process significantly. Even damage to skin that is vulnerable to leg ulcer development can bring on the condition.

Do not expose your legs to strong heat sources - this is a common mistake as people often think heat will help circulation. Instead, the heat can damage skin and veins.

Try to arrange your home so that it is as accident free as possible. Get rid of protruding objects, make sure the floors are not slippery and so on. See the check list.

3. DON'T CROSS YOUR LEGS

When sitting or lying down do not cross your legs. It can reduce circulation and therefore worsen the venous problems.

4. AVOID WEARING RESTRICTIVE CLOTHING

Tight pants, tight socks, garters or anything that can restrict blood flow must be avoided. It is difficult to estimate what damage can be caused but as a general rule this should not be too disruptive to your dress plans - there are many alternatives you can plan for.

5. MAINTAIN GOOD HYGIENE & INFECTION CONTROL

If you are involved with dressing changes or any activity around the leg ulcer make sure you have washed your hands thoroughly and follow your instructions accurately. An infection caused by unclean hands can seriously set you back as far as the healing process is concerned. Check with your nurse as to what procedures should be followed if you have any doubts at all. Make sure you know the early warning signs of an infection and if you suspect a problem seek medical help immediately.

6. AVOID SCRATCHING

This is the most common way of bringing on a leg ulcer by your own actions. Often scratching can be due to dry itchy skin and there are products available that can rectify this. You may scratch without thinking so make sure your nails are kept short to minimize damage.

7. TRAVEL TIPS

When riding in the car, stop, get out and walk around frequently to avoid build-up of fluid in the legs.

If you sit for a long period of time in the same position on an airplane, try to get up and walk about or do the foot exercises shown. Informing the attendant of your needs may help you obtain a seat with more leg room or better access to the aisle.

8. AVOIDING DIRECT SOURCES OF HEAT

Any source of heat --- fires, the sun, Jacuzzis, saunas, hot tubs help the veins dilate. You must avoid these or use with extreme caution to avoid further damaging of the veins.

SELF ASSESSMENT CHECKLIST
tick any you need to action

Premier Self Help Tips

Compression ☐

Exercise ☐

Leg elevation ☐

Adherence to treatment ☐

Compression stockings ☐

Skin care ☐

Pain relief ☐

Lifestyle Tips

Quitting smoking ☐

Nutrition ☐

Weight loss ☐

Family / caregiver support ☐

Positive attitude ☐

Common Sense Tips

Avoid standing ☐

Do no harm ☐

Avoid crossing legs ☐

Avoid restrictive clothing ☐

No scratching ☐

Avoid direct heat ☐

Good hygiene ☐

Travel tips ☐

GETTING IT ALL INTO PERSPECTIVE

The root cause of venous leg ulcers is the swelling of the legs caused by high venous blood pressure. Prevent the swelling and you are controlling the disease. This means that for most people the most important aspect of treatment and prevention is effective compression of the legs through bandaging or stockings.

Although all the self help tips and adherence to treatment actioned by the patient are vital for healing and prevention, the morale and well being of the patient is also very important.

Caregivers, family members and medical staff should listen, nurture and communicate effectively and always ensure any pain issue is addressed.

Finally the patient has to take some ownership of the treatment by way of being assertive, asking questions and making sure there is understanding. There are many players in the medical team and the only way to ensure success is for the patient to be the major player in the winning team.